NIACINAMIDE FOR BEGINNERS

Unlocking Radiant Skin And Optimal Health, A Comprehensive Guide To Niacinamide's Benefits, Uses, Transformational Power, And Overall Vitality

Georgette Lockett

DISCLAIMER

The author of this book is not affiliated, associated, endorsed, sponsored, or approved by any company or individual. The views and opinions expressed in this book are solely those of the author and do not necessarily reflect the official policy or position of any entity.

The author hereby disclaims any relationship, collaboration, or partnership with any company or individual mentioned in this book. Any references to products, services, or individuals are provided for informational purposes only and should not be construed as an endorsement or recommendation.

Readers are advised to exercise their own judgment and discretion when applying the information provided in this book. The author shall not be held responsible for any actions taken by readers based on the content of this book.

This book is intended for general informational purposes only, and the author makes no representations or warranties of any kind, express or implied, about the completeness, accuracy, reliability, suitability, or availability of the information contained herein. Any reliance on the information in this book is at the reader's own risk.

The author reserves the right to update, change, or modify any information in this book without notice. It is the responsibility of the reader to verify any information before taking any actions based on the content of this book.

By reading this book, the reader acknowledges and agrees to the terms of this disclaimer.

Table of Contents

INTRODUCTION

Skincare fans often traverse a maze of substances, each offering a different set of advantages. Niacinamide stands out as a versatile and scientifically acknowledged chemical among them. Understanding the relevance of skincare components and digging into Niacinamide's details elucidates its critical function in skincare regimens.

Importance Of Skincare Ingredients

The skin, being the body's biggest organ, needs meticulous care and attention. Skincare components are essential for fostering and preserving skin health. They are the foundation of skincare products, providing a wide range of benefits from hydration and protection to rejuvenation and healing.

Niacinamide, for example, provides diverse benefits by addressing a variety of skin issues such as hyperpigmentation, acne, fine wrinkles, and dullness. These chemicals' effectiveness is supported by scientific studies, making them more than just marketing buzzwords but established agents of skin change.

Overview Of Niacinamide

Niacinamide, commonly known as nicotinamide or Vitamin B3, is a water-soluble vitamin that is gaining popularity in the beauty business. It is notable for its flexibility and compatibility with many skin types, particularly sensitive skin.

This substance has a plethora of advantages, including the capacity to strengthen the skin's barrier function, control oil production, and reduce the visibility of pores. It's also known for its anti-inflammatory effects, making it a good option for soothing inflamed skin and reducing redness.

Purpose And Scope Of The Guide

This tutorial aims to dispel myths about Niacinamide by offering in-depth information on its qualities, methods of action, and use in skincare regimens. This book seeks to enable consumers to make educated choices about including Niacinamide in their skincare routine by covering its numerous features, from scientific research to practical use.

1. **Benefits and Mechanisms:** Uncovering the many benefits of Niacinamide and explaining how it works on a cellular level to help the skin.

2. **Suitability for particular Skin Concerns:** Discuss how Niacinamide handles particular skin concerns such as hyperpigmentation, acne, and aging symptoms, among others.

3. **Skincare Routine Integration:** Advice on incorporating Niacinamide into skincare regimens,

compatibility with other substances, and possible synergy.

4. Myths & misunderstandings: Addressing common myths or misunderstandings about Niacinamide to bring clarification and eliminate uncertainty.

5. Potential adverse Effects and measures: Highlighting any potential adverse effects and recommending measures for safe use.

In summary, this book strives to be a thorough resource, providing skincare aficionados with the information needed to fully use Niacinamide's potential for healthier, more radiant skin.

CHAPTER 1

What Is Niacinamide?

Definition And Composition

Niacinamide, commonly known as nicotinamide or Vitamin B3, is a water-soluble vitamin that is an essential component of the B-complex family. It has a similar molecular structure to niacin (nicotinic acid), however, they have different characteristics. Niacinamide has the chemical formula $C_6H_6N_2O$ and is made up of a pyridine ring with a carboxamide group (-$CONH_2$) attached.

As an essential vitamin for human health, niacinamide is involved in a variety of physiological activities such as energy metabolism, DNA repair, and cell signaling. Because of its possible skin advantages, such as enhancing texture, decreasing inflammation, and correcting hyperpigmentation, it is often utilized in skincare and cosmetic products.

Historical Background

Niacinamide's history begins with the discovery of niacin, its predecessor, in the early twentieth century. Niacin has been found as an important role in the prevention and treatment of pellagra, a condition that causes dermatitis, diarrhea, and dementia. Later, researchers discovered that niacinamide, a niacin derivative, also has therapeutic qualities.

The link between niacin and pellagra was especially relevant in the early twentieth century when public health initiatives targeted addressing nutritional inadequacies. As scientists investigated their roles and activities inside the body, the difference between niacin and niacinamide became apparent.

Sources And Production

Niacinamide is naturally available in a variety of food sources, making it a vital dietary component. Niacinamide-rich foods include meat, fish, poultry, nuts, seeds, and some vegetables. Furthermore, the body may convert niacin (nicotinic acid) into niacinamide via enzymatic mechanisms, guaranteeing a consistent supply of this vital vitamin.

In terms of manufacture, niacinamide may be created chemically or extracted from natural sources. Chemical processes are used to convert precursor chemicals into niacinamide. Natural sources, on the other hand, provide an alternate way for niacinamide extraction or separation from organic components.

Niacinamide manufacture for cosmetic and skincare purposes often includes high-quality manufacturing techniques to assure purity and effectiveness. Niacinamide is a popular option in the creation of many skincare products due to its stability and compatibility with other components, which contributes to its extensive usage in the beauty industry.

To summarize, niacinamide is a versatile chemical with a long history of use in the treatment of nutritional deficiencies. Its definition, composition, historical history, sources, and production all contribute to a thorough grasp of this crucial nutrient and its many uses.

CHAPTER 2

Benefits Of Niacinamide

Skin Health And Functionality

Niacinamide, commonly known as vitamin B3 or nicotinamide, is a water-soluble vitamin that is essential for skin health and functioning. Because of its numerous qualities that contribute to total skin well-being, its multiple advantages have attracted attention in dermatology and skincare.

1. Niacinamide plays an important part in enhancing the skin's barrier function. The skin's barrier, which is mostly made up of lipids, acts as a protection against environmental aggressors, moisture loss, and toxic chemicals. Niacinamide contributes to the maintenance of this barrier by lowering transepidermal water loss (TEWL) and strengthening the skin's resistance to external stresses.

2. Moisturization: Because of its potential to increase the moisture content of the skin, niacinamide is a prominent component in skincare formulations. By increasing the synthesis of ceramides, a kind of lipid important for moisture retention, it helps to keep the skin moisturized and supple, which is essential for maintaining a healthy skin look.

3. Anti-Inflammatory Properties: Niacinamide has anti-inflammatory properties, making it useful for those who have sensitive or inflammatory skin disorders like acne, rosacea, or eczema. It helps to reduce redness, soothe irritated skin, and maybe decrease inflammatory reactions.

4. Niacinamide may help manage sebum production in those who have oily or acne-prone skin. It may help manage acne and reduce the appearance of enlarged pores by controlling oil secretion.

Role In Skincare Regimens

Because of its flexibility and compatibility with many skin types, niacinamide has found a place in many skincare programs. Because of its formulation stability and compatibility with other active ingredients, it is an appealing option for both preventative and remedial skincare treatments.

1. Niacinamide is compatible with a wide range of skincare components, including retinoids, antioxidants, hyaluronic acid, and alpha hydroxy acids, without generating adverse reactions. Because of its flexibility, it may be used in a variety of skincare products such as serums, moisturizers, and toners, boosting their overall effectiveness.

2. **Preventive and Corrective:** Because niacinamide is adaptable, it may be taken as a preventive strategy to maintain healthy skin or as a corrective remedy to address particular difficulties.

Its ability to address many skin concerns makes it an important complement to everyday skincare regimes.

Scientific Evidence And Studies

An increasing collection of scientific research and clinical investigations backs up niacinamide's usefulness in skin care.

1. **Acne Management:** Studies have shown that niacinamide is excellent in treating acne. Its anti-inflammatory characteristics may help minimize acne lesions and lower sebum production, making it a viable acne treatment alternative.

2. **Hyperpigmentation:** Niacinamide's potential to reduce hyperpigmentation has been studied. It may help to reduce the appearance of dark spots, melasma, and uneven skin tone by blocking melanin synthesis and improving skin texture, according to research.

3. **Anti-aging:** Studies have been conducted to investigate the impact of niacinamide in treating the indications of aging. It has shown promise in reducing the appearance of fine lines, wrinkles, and elasticity by promoting collagen formation and keeping the skin hydrated.

Finally, niacinamide is a flexible and evidence-based skincare component, providing a range of benefits ranging from strengthening skin barrier function to treating numerous skin issues. Its use in skincare regimens emphasizes its importance in supporting overall skin health and vitality.

CHAPTER 3

How Niacinamide Works

Niacinamide, commonly known as Vitamin B3 or nicotinamide, is a versatile and multifunctional chemical important for skin health. Understanding how niacinamide works at the molecular level sheds light on its many skincare advantages.

Mechanism Of Action In Skin

Niacinamide works on the skin via complex metabolic mechanisms. One important method is that it is converted to nicotinamide adenine dinucleotide (NAD+), a vital coenzyme involved in a variety of cellular functions. NAD+ is required for energy synthesis, DNA repair, and signaling pathways that control cell survival and function.

In the context of skincare, replenishing NAD+ levels with niacinamide aids cellular metabolism, resulting in increased skin vibrancy and resilience.

Furthermore, niacinamide has been proven to increase the creation of essential structural proteins such as collagen and keratin, hence increasing skin firmness and elasticity.

Furthermore, niacinamide has a role in the control of inflammatory processes. It regulates the action of inflammatory mediators like cytokines, assisting in the maintenance of a balanced inflammatory response in the skin. This anti-inflammatory activity is especially useful in the treatment of acne and rosacea, where excessive inflammation leads to skin problems.

Absorption And Bioavailability

Niacinamide has a high level of skin penetration and bioavailability. When administered topically, it may easily penetrate the stratum corneum, the skin's outermost layer, and reach the deeper levels where it exerts its biological effects.

Niacinamide's fast absorption makes it a suitable component for topical skincare formulations.

Niacinamide's bioavailability guarantees that it may exercise its effects in a focused way. Niacinamide, once absorbed, may modify cellular activity in the skin without creating irritation or sensitivity, making it suited for a variety of skin types, including sensitive and reactive skin.

Interaction With Other Skincare Ingredients

Niacinamide has been shown to complement and improve the effectiveness of a variety of cosmetic products. It may be used together with other active components in skincare regimes without sacrificing stability or creating unwanted effects.

For example, niacinamide collaborates with antioxidants like vitamin C to give increased protection against oxidative stress. This mixture aids in the neutralization of free radicals, therefore improving general skin health and avoiding premature aging.

Furthermore, niacinamide enhances the activity of substances such as retinoids. While retinoids concentrate on cell turnover and collagen formation, niacinamide helps to maintain a healthy skin barrier, reducing possible adverse effects such as dryness or irritation associated with retinoid usage.

Finally, knowing the processes by which niacinamide functions in the skin provides insight into its many advantages and compatibility with different skincare formulas. Niacinamide is a key tool in supporting general skin health and treating particular skincare issues due to its ability to promote cellular processes, reduce inflammation, and work synergistically with other substances.

CHAPTER 4

Niacinamide For Various Skin Types

Effects On Different Skin Types (Dry, Oily, Sensitive, Etc.)

1. Dry skin:

• Moisture Retention: Niacinamide improves moisture retention by strengthening the skin barrier.

• Improved Texture: It improves the skin's natural lipid barrier, resulting in smoother and softer skin.

2. Oily Skin:

• Sebum Regulation: Niacinamide controls sebum production, lowering oiliness without overdrying the skin.

• Pore Minimization: Because of its capacity to control sebum, it may also aid in reducing the appearance of enlarged pores.

3. Skin Sensitive:

• Calming qualities: Niacinamide has anti-inflammatory qualities that help to reduce redness and irritation.

• Barrier Repair: It fortifies the skin's barrier, making it more resistant to irritants.

4. Skin Type: Combination

• Balancing: Niacinamide may help balance both oily and dry parts of mixed skin, delivering moisture without producing undue oiliness.

Addressing Specific Skin Concerns (Acne, Aging, Hyperpigmentation, Etc.)

1. Acne:

• Sebum Regulation: Niacinamide reduces acne outbreaks by decreasing sebum production.

•   Anti-inflammatory: Its anti-inflammatory characteristics may help reduce acne-related redness and irritation.

2. Aging:

• Collagen production: Niacinamide promotes collagen production, resulting in firmer, more elastic skin and a reduction in the appearance of fine lines and wrinkles.

• Antioxidant Properties: It protects against oxidative stress, which is a major cause of premature aging.

3. Hyperpigmentation:

• Even Skin Tone: Niacinamide prevents melanin transport to skin cells, which helps to reduce the appearance of dark patches and hyperpigmentation.

• Brightening: By controlling melanin synthesis, it helps to get a more luminous and even complexion.

Usage Recommendations

• **Concentration:** Products generally include niacinamide at concentrations ranging from 2% to 10%, making them suited for a variety of skin types.

• Use it regularly, either in the morning or at night, depending on personal choice.

Concerns And Compatibility

• **Niacinamide Interactions:** Niacinamide is typically well-tolerated and compatible with a wide range of other skincare products, including retinoids, hyaluronic acid, and antioxidants.

• **PH Consideration:** Because it thrives in a broad pH range, it is adaptable and suitable with the majority of skincare products.

Niacinamide's adaptability makes it a notable component for a variety of skin types and issues, providing a holistic approach to skincare with its numerous advantages.

Consultation with a dermatologist or skincare specialist may help you tailor its use to your unique skin requirements.

CHAPTER 5

Niacinamide In Cosmetics And Skincare Products

Niacinamide, commonly known as vitamin B3 or nicotinamide, has received a lot of attention in the cosmetic and skincare industry because of its many skin health advantages. In this chapter, we will look at the formulations and concentrations of niacinamide in skincare products, how to choose the proper product, and how to use it.

Formulations And Concentrations

Niacinamide is a water-soluble vitamin that may be used in a variety of forms. It is found in a variety of skincare products like creams, serums, lotions, and even cleansers. Because of niacinamide's flexibility, formulators may combine it into a variety of products to target particular skin conditions.

Niacinamide concentrations in skincare products may vary, and customers need to read the labeling. Concentrations typically vary from 2% to 10%, with 5% being a popular and effective quantity in many formulations. Higher doses may be available in more specialized products, but to prevent any side effects, it is important to follow product instructions and contact skincare specialists.

Choosing The Right Product

When choosing a niacinamide-containing product, keep your skin type, problems, and entire skincare regimen in mind. Niacinamide is well-known for being compatible with a wide range of skin types, including sensitive and acne-prone skin.

Look for niacinamide products that include additional helpful compounds like hyaluronic acid, antioxidants, and peptides. These combinations may improve the product's overall efficacy and give a more holistic approach to skincare.

Take note of the product's packaging as well. Airtight and opaque containers may help maintain niacinamide's stability and effectiveness by shielding it from deterioration caused by light and air exposure.

Application Methods

Niacinamide is simple to include in your skincare regimen, and its flexibility allows for a variety of application techniques. Here are some typical methods to include niacinamide in your beauty routine:

1. Serums:

• Niacinamide serums are popular due to their concentrated compositions, which allow them to effectively treat certain skin issues. They are usually used after cleansing but before moisturizing.

2. Moisturizers:

• Niacinamide-infused moisturizers give moisture as well as vitamin benefits. These are appropriate for everyday usage and may be used in the morning and evening.

3. Creams:

• Niacinamide creams are heavier formulations that are good for dry or older skin. They may be used as part of a nighttime skincare regimen.

4. Treatments for Spots:

• Niacinamide spot treatments are available for the focused treatment of certain skin issues. For more targeted outcomes, they are administered specifically to troubled regions.

5. Cleansers:

• Some face cleansers include niacinamide to deliver its advantages while cleaning.

These are excellent for everyday usage and provide a mild introduction to niacinamide.

It's critical to incorporate niacinamide into your skincare regimen gradually, particularly if you're already utilizing other active components. Patch testing may assist in verifying compatibility and reduce discomfort.

Finally, knowing the formulations, concentrations, and application techniques of niacinamide in cosmetics and skin care products enables customers to make educated decisions that address their individual skin requirements and concerns. To get the full advantages of niacinamide, like with any skincare component, persistence and patience are required.

CHAPTER 6

Safety And Side Effects

Recommended Dosages

Niacinamide, a kind of vitamin B3, is usually regarded as safe when taken at suitable levels. Dosages for oral supplements generally vary from 250 to 500 mg per day. These dosages are often used to treat a variety of health issues, including skin problems, arthritis, and diabetes. However, since individual requirements and tolerances differ, it is critical to speak with a healthcare expert before beginning any supplementation routine.

Niacinamide concentrations in skincare products typically vary from 2% to 10%. It's crucial to remember that larger concentrations don't automatically imply more efficacy, since efficacy is frequently dependent on formulation, skin type, and total product composition.

Potential Adverse Reactions

Niacinamide is typically well tolerated by the majority of people. It usually has fewer negative effects than niacin (another kind of vitamin B3), such as flushing or itching. However, some people may have mild side effects such as:

1. **Skin Irritation:** Although uncommon, some people may suffer redness, itching, or irritation when using niacinamide-containing skincare products, particularly at higher concentrations or in conjunction with other active components.

2. **Allergic Reactions:** Although allergic reactions to niacinamide are uncommon, they are possible. Rashes, itching, swelling, and trouble breathing are all possible symptoms. If any serious allergic reactions develop, seek medical assistance immediately.

Precautions And Contradictions

Despite its largely positive safety profile, the following precautions should be taken:

1. Individuals with severely sensitive or allergic-prone skin should do patch tests before using niacinamide-containing products. This allows you to analyze any negative responses before applying the product to a bigger area.

2. **Interaction with Other Skincare Products:** Niacinamide is a generally stable component that is compatible with a wide range of skincare products. However, there have been concerns regarding possible interactions when taken in conjunction with some acidic formulations, such as those containing vitamin C. According to some sources, when combined at extremely low pH values, they may destabilize each other. More study is required, however, to determine the magnitude of these interactions and their influence on efficacy.

3. Pregnancy and nursing: There is little evidence that niacinamide supplementation is safe during pregnancy and nursing. Pregnant and nursing women should check with their doctor before taking niacinamide supplements or high-concentration skincare products.

4. Underlying Medical issues: People with pre-existing medical issues or those on medicines should speak with their doctor before using niacinamide supplements to avoid any possible interactions or side effects.

When used correctly, whether in dietary supplements or cosmetic products, niacinamide is typically safe for most people. While bad reactions are uncommon, it is critical to patch-test new skincare products and speak with a healthcare practitioner, particularly if you have pre-existing medical issues or are pregnant or nursing.

CHAPTER 7

Incorporating Niacinamide Into Your Skincare Routine

Step-By-Step Guide For Usage

1. To remove pollutants and makeup, begin with a mild cleanser suitable to your skin type. This helps your skin absorb the following products more effectively.

2. **Toning (Optional):** Some people like to apply a toner to adjust the pH levels of their skin. While not required, if you use a toner, make sure it is alcohol-free to avoid drying out your skin.

3. **Niacinamide Application:** Cover your whole face with a pea-sized dollop of niacinamide serum or cream. Massage it into your skin in upward strokes until it is completely absorbed. Follow the product's frequency directions (typically morning and night).

4. **Moisturization:** Apply a moisturizer to lock in the benefits of niacinamide. This aids in keeping the skin hydrated.

5. **Sun Protection:** Always conclude your day with a broad-spectrum sunscreen with an SPF of 30 or higher to protect your skin from damaging UV radiation.

Combining Niacinamide With Other Skincare Ingredients

• **Vitamin C:** These two chemicals complement each other effectively in terms of brightening and leveling out skin tone. To prevent possible interactions, take vitamin C in the morning and niacinamide in the evening.

• **Hyaluronic Acid:** Niacinamide may supplement hyaluronic acid's moisturizing capabilities, providing a balance between moisture retention and general skin health.

- **Retinoids:** Niacinamide may help reduce the irritation produced by retinoids. Allow niacinamide to absorb before proceeding with retinoids.

- **AHAs/BHAs:** Using niacinamide in conjunction with alpha hydroxy acids (AHAs) or beta hydroxy acids (BHAs) may improve exfoliation and regulate sebum production. However, some people may be sensitive to these components, thus a patch test is recommended before mixing them.

Tips For Optimal Results

1. **Patch Test:** Before adding a new niacinamide product or combining it with other active substances, do a patch test to verify no adverse reactions occur.

2. Niacinamide has cumulative effects over time, thus continuous usage is necessary for maximum outcomes.

3. If you're new to niacinamide or mixing it with other actives, start with lesser concentrations and gradually increase frequency or potency as your skin adjusts.

4. **Consult a specialist:** If you're unsure how to include niacinamide into your regimen or if you have particular skin issues, get specialized counsel from a dermatologist or skincare specialist.

Keep in mind that everyone's skin is unique, so what works for one person may not work for another. To get the greatest effects from niacinamide, customize your skincare regimen depending on your skin type, issues, and tolerance levels.

CHAPTER 8

The Science Behind Niacinamide

Research Findings And Clinical Trials

Niacinamide, commonly known as vitamin B3 or nicotinamide, has received a lot of interest in the scientific community owing to its wide variety of possible skin health advantages. Numerous research results and clinical studies have offered insights into niacinamide's processes and effects.

Action Mechanisms:

1. Anti-Inflammatory Effects:

• According to research, niacinamide has significant anti-inflammatory qualities. It works by suppressing the inflammatory mediators implicated in numerous skin problems, making it an invaluable tool in the treatment of inflammatory skin disorders such as acne and rosacea.

2. Collagen Production:

• Research has shown that niacinamide stimulates collagen production in the skin. Because collagen is essential for preserving skin elasticity and firmness, niacinamide is a significant ingredient in anti-aging products.

3. Melanin Control:

• Niacinamide has been demonstrated to modulate melanin synthesis, making it useful for treating hyperpigmentation concerns including dark patches and melasma. This process helps to explain why it's so popular in skin brightening and skin tone-evening products.

4. Enhancement of Barrier Function:

• The vitamin B3 derivative supports the skin's natural barrier function.

Niacinamide helps prevent water loss by increasing the skin barrier, making it advantageous for those with dry or sensitive skin.

Clinical Research:

1. Acne Treatment:

• Clinical investigations have shown that niacinamide is useful in treating acne. Its anti-inflammatory effects, together with its ability to regulate sebum, make it an important component of acne treatment regimens.

2. Anti-Aging Properties:

• Research on the effects of niacinamide on aging skin has shown improvements in fine lines, wrinkles, and general skin texture. Its capacity to increase collagen formation adds to its anti-aging properties.

3. Reducing Hyperpigmentation:

• Hyperpigmentation clinical studies have emphasized niacinamide's effectiveness in decreasing the appearance of dark patches and uneven skin tone. This has resulted in its use in formulations addressing hyperpigmentation concerns.

Future Potential And Ongoing Studies

Niacinamide is still being studied scientifically, with research looking at its possible uses and methods of action. Among the topics of interest are:

1. Neuroprotective Properties:

• A new study reveals that niacinamide may have neuroprotective properties, implying a larger range of advantages beyond skincare. Its significance in neurodegenerative disorders is being studied further.

2. Photoprotection:

• Niacinamide has shown potential in terms of UV (ultraviolet) radiation protection. Ongoing research seeks to learn more about its photoprotective mechanisms and prospective uses in sunscreens and other protective compositions.

3. Therapies in Combination:

• Researchers are researching niacinamide's synergistic benefits when paired with other skincare components. Combinations including antioxidants, retinoids, and peptides are being investigated for improved skincare results.

Expert Opinions And Insights

Leading dermatologists and skincare specialists have shared useful information about the usage of niacinamide:

- "Niacinamide is a versatile ingredient with a proven safety record." Its ability to address multiple skin concerns, coupled with minimal side effects, makes it a favorite among both dermatologists and skincare enthusiasts."

PhD Skincare Scientist Professor:

- "The scientific literature on niacinamide is extensive and expanding." Its multifaceted benefits and compatibility with various skin types make it a valuable asset in the development of innovative skincare formulations."

Finally, the science underpinning niacinamide emphasizes its usefulness in skin care, as shown by rigorous study results and current studies. Niacinamide is anticipated to continue playing a crucial role in the expanding landscape of skincare research as our knowledge of its actions increases.

CHAPTER 9

Niacinamide In Health And Beyond Skincare

Other Applications In Health And Wellness

Cardiovascular Fitness

While nicotinamide, commonly known as niacinamide, is well-known for its function in skincare, its advantages go beyond dermatology. According to research, niacinamide may have a role in enhancing cardiovascular health. Niacinamide is a precursor to nicotinamide adenine dinucleotide (NAD), a coenzyme required for many cellular functions, including those related to cardiovascular function.

Niacinamide has been studied for its potential in the treatment of cardiovascular disease. It is hypothesized that its capacity to boost NAD synthesis influences cellular energy metabolism, possibly affecting heart function. However, although early results are encouraging, further study is required to establish conclusive correlations between niacinamide consumption and cardiovascular outcomes.

Cognitive Ability

The involvement of niacinamide in cellular energy metabolism raises concerns regarding its possible influence on cognitive function. The brain is very energy-dependent, and sufficient NAD levels are required for neuronal function. According to some research, niacinamide may benefit cognitive function by assisting brain cells in meeting their energy needs.

While research on niacinamide's cognitive advantages is still in its early stages, experts are looking into its potential to prevent age-related cognitive decline and neurodegenerative diseases.

It's a promising option for incorporating niacinamide into larger health and wellness programs.

Immune System Aid

Niacinamide is known for its immunomodulatory effects. NAD, formed from niacinamide, is involved in a variety of immunological responses. Preclinical research has shown that niacinamide can regulate immune cell activity, which might have consequences for maintaining a healthy immune system.

This research looks at the function of niacinamide in immune cell activation, inflammation modulation, and general immune system control. However, these findings should be interpreted with care since the translation of preclinical data to human health needs more research.

Emerging Uses And Developments

Metabolic Fitness

A new study indicates a possible relationship between niacinamide and metabolic health. NAD, which is controlled by niacinamide, is an important factor in cellular energy metabolism. Some research suggests that niacinamide supplementation may benefit metabolic diseases such as insulin resistance and type 2 diabetes.

This field of investigation is quite promising, but it needs significant clinical confirmation. Understanding how niacinamide affects metabolic pathways might lead to novel approaches to treating metabolic diseases and improving general health.

Antioxidant and Anti-Inflammatory Activity

Niacinamide is gaining popularity for its antioxidant and anti-inflammatory qualities, in addition to its proven function in skincare.

These properties may have larger health consequences, notably in the treatment of oxidative stress and chronic inflammation.

The ongoing study is looking at niacinamide's ability to reduce oxidative damage and inflammation in different tissues, with implications for anything from arthritis to neurological illnesses. Niacinamide may find uses in treatments focused on moderating oxidative and inflammatory processes as knowledge advances.

Niacinamide In Alternative Fields

Dietary Supplements and Nutraceuticals

Niacinamide has found a position in the domain of nutraceuticals and dietary supplements as our awareness of its health advantages grows. Niacinamide pills are growing more popular as customers strive to maximize their potential for both skincare and general well-being.

Niacinamide supplement formulation includes considerations for bioavailability, dose, and possible interactions with other substances. Niacinamide is being positioned as a vital component of supplement regimens as interest in preventative health and holistic well-being develops.

Complementary and Alternative Medicine

Practitioners in integrative medicine are investigating the inclusion of niacinamide into holistic therapeutic practices. Its diverse significance in cellular processes, along with its low toxicity, makes it a promising choice for integrative health techniques.

Integrative medicine tries to mix traditional and alternative treatments, and niacinamide's adaptability makes it a potential asset in treating a wide range of health issues. Collaboration between conventional healthcare doctors and alternative medicine practitioners may help to better investigate niacinamide's integrative potential.

Niacinamide's evolution from a skincare mainstay to a versatile health contributor demonstrates its adaptability and significance in a variety of physiological processes. As continuous research reveals new aspects of niacinamide's potential, it offers promise not just for skincare lovers but also for anyone looking for holistic health and well-being solutions. However, it is critical to approach emergent applications with a balanced mindset, realizing the need for more rigorous scientific research to properly understand and evaluate these potential advantages.

CHAPTER 10

Exploring Niacinamide Myths And Misconceptions

Common Myths Debunked

1. Myth: Niacinamide, like Niacin, causes skin flushing:

• Niacinamide and niacin (nicotinic acid) are linked, but their effects vary. Because of its effect on blood artery dilatation, niacin may induce flushing, redness, or warmth of the skin. Niacinamide, on the other hand, does not produce flushing because it does not affect prostaglandin production in the same manner as niacin does.

2. Myth: It's ineffective because it lacks active ingredients:

• Fact: Despite not being as visually appealing as some other skincare ingredients, niacinamide is a powerful multitasker. It works quietly yet efficiently on a variety of skin issues, including texture, enlarged pores, dullness, and pigmentation.

3. Myth: Niacinamide and Vitamin C Shouldn't Be Mixed:

• Fact: This myth emerged as a result of worries about their probable interplay in the formation of niacin. However, research has shown that mixing niacinamide with vitamin C does not result in the synthesis of niacin on the skin. Both may complement one other's effects and function well together.

4. Myth: Niacinamide causes skin thinning or sensitivity:

• Fact: Niacinamide is well tolerated by the majority of skin types. In actuality, it strengthens the skin barrier, increasing its resilience and maybe lowering sensitivity, redness, and irritation.

Clarifying Misinformation

1. Niacinamide Doesn't Produce Visible Results:

• Clarification: While niacinamide does not work miracles overnight, persistent usage may lead to considerable changes in skin texture, tone, and appearance. Its advantages may take time to develop, but they are often obvious.

2. All Niacinamide Products Are the Same, According to the Manufacturer:

• Clarification: Niacinamide comes in a variety of forms and concentrations, which affects its effectiveness and compatibility with different skin types. Their performance is influenced by factors such as formulation quality, pH levels, and extra additives.

3. High Concentrations Produce Better Results:

• Clarification: Niacinamide is beneficial at a variety of concentrations ranging from 2% to 10%. Higher concentrations may not always provide better outcomes and may cause discomfort in those with sensitive skin.

Empowering Informed Decision-Making

Understanding the science behind Niacinamide allows you to make more educated choices regarding your skincare regimen. Knowing its advantages, limits, and potential interactions may help people choose products that are right for their skin. Individuals with unique skin issues or disorders should seek specialized guidance from skincare specialists or dermatologists.

Education is essential for dispelling myths and misunderstandings about Niacinamide. Individuals may easily add this versatile substance into their skincare routine and get its many advantages by equipping themselves with appropriate knowledge.

Conclusion

Niacinamide, commonly known as Vitamin B3 or nicotinamide, is a unique molecule that has made tremendous advances in cosmetics, health, and well-being. This adaptable nutrient has risen in popularity because of its many advantages and broad uses in a variety of fields.

Recap Of Key Takeaways

Throughout our research, we discovered Niacinamide's several benefits. It is a key element in skincare, capable of addressing a wide range of skin issues. Niacinamide's effectiveness has been shown over and again, from improving skin barrier function and lowering inflammation to controlling sebum production and eliminating hyperpigmentation. Because of its usefulness in promoting general skin health, it is a key component of many skincare formulas.

The science underlying Niacinamide shows its complex modes of action, which include improving cellular metabolism and influencing several biochemical processes in the skin. Because of its absorption and bioavailability, it is a steady and dependable component in skincare products, assuring its efficacy when administered topically.

Future Trends And Developments In Niacinamide

Niacinamide's future shows promise in several areas. Continued research and clinical trials may reveal additional facets of its efficacy, perhaps leading to the discovery of innovative uses in skincare and beyond. Innovations in formulation technology may improve its delivery methods, improving penetration and effectiveness in treating a variety of skin issues.

Furthermore, the importance of niacinamide in health and well-being is growing beyond cosmetics.

Its potential for treating ailments such as arthritis, diabetes, and neurological disorders is being investigated, demonstrating that its value extends beyond cosmetic uses.

As time goes on, including Niacinamide in skincare regimes and researching its potential in numerous health areas is not only smart but also promising. Choosing trustworthy products with suitable Niacinamide concentrations, taking into account individual skin sensitivities, and consulting with skincare specialists for individualized guidance are all recommendations for effective use.

Finally, the exploration of Niacinamide shows a formidable ally in skincare and wellness, with its adaptability and efficacy making it a useful asset. Understanding its mechanics, recognizing its advantages, and embracing its potential pave the way for a bright future in cosmetic and therapeutic applications.

Niacinamide's path has been one of continuous discovery and invention, presenting a plethora of options and advantages for those seeking better skin and exploring new avenues in healthcare.

THE END

www.ingramcontent.com/pod-product-compliance
Lightning Source LLC
Chambersburg PA
CBHW050749260726
48661CB00001B/498